Hey Caregiver

DEVOTIONAL & PRAYER JOURNAL

*To Strengthen, Empower, and Inspire Caregivers
to Keep Going, Keep Pushing, Keep Loving and
Keep CARING!*

PRISCILLA J. JEAN-LOUIS

FOUNDER OF MY FAVORITE GIRL & ALZHEIMER'S

"Greater love has no one than this: to lay down one's life for one's friends." *John 15:13 NIV*

Hey Caregiver

This **Devotional & Prayer Journal** is dedicated to my mother, **Vera M. Johnson,** who I affectionately call "*My Favorite Girl.*" Thank you for teaching me how to care deeply for others with no motive but a heart full of love. You are my greatest example of what it means to truly care. I will always be honored that God chose me to care for you in your later days. I love you, girl!

To my grandmother by love, **Julie M. Powell**—thank you for choosing me and loving me as if I were your own. It was my deepest honor to care for you during the last five years of your life. We miss you so much. On January 29, 2022, at 12:09 p.m., **#LOVEWon.**

Lastly, to **every person who selflessly lays down their life each day to care for a loved one,** this is dedicated to you.

The journey of a caregiver is not an easy one. It is filled with twists and turns, steep climbs and deep valleys. There will be days when the weight feels unbearable—when walking away feels like the only option. Don't.

It is my heartfelt prayer that on those difficult days, you will reach for this devotional and find the strength you need to take the next step. That the prayers within these pages—and the ones you pour out from your own heart—will breathe fresh courage into your spirit and give you the fortitude to **Keep Going. Keep Pushing. Keep Loving. Keep Caring.**

You are not alone. I see you. I honor you. I love you—and I'm praying for you.

Acknowledgements

Kaylin, I'm so grateful for you. Thank you for sticking this caregiving journey out with me—without ever complaining. You pushed me to get started with my books... here's the first one!

Destiny Nicole, I'm grateful to be your mom. You are one of the greatest parts of me. You're a true "Granny Girl," and she would be so proud of the work you're doing.

To My Village – Tara, Danette, Pastors Gerald & Judy Mandrell, Pastor Tee, Carolyn, Khalilah, Shynira, Olivia, Paula, Zemoria, Brenda, Vanessa, Anna, Jessi, Saralyn, Grandma DK, Pastors Thomas "Pop" and Dorothy Colbert—THANK YOU! Thank you for praying for me, pushing me, showing up for me, and simply loving me. Thank you for caring for the caregiver!

Contents

Contents

Journal

If it concerns you, it concerns God.

Loving to the End

Before the Passover celebration, Jesus knew that his hour had come to leave this world and return to his Father. He had loved his disciples during his ministry on earth, and now he loved them to the very end. John 13:1 NLT

Caregiving is one of the purest expressions of love. It's a love that shows up when it's inconvenient, continues when it's exhausting, and stays even when there's no applause. This is the kind of love Jesus demonstrated when He knelt to wash His disciples' feet and prepared to face the cross.

"Having loved his own who were in the world, he loved them to the end.
– John 13:1 NIV

Jesus didn't stop loving when it got hard. He didn't withdraw when His disciples were imperfect. Instead, He loved fully and faithfully—right to the end.

As caregivers, we are called into this sacred work of love. It's not always easy. There are days when exhaustion whispers, "You've done enough." There are moments when frustration clouds our patience. Yet, even in those moments, we can draw strength from the One who never stops loving us.

Jesus shows us that caregiving is not just about meeting needs; it's about honoring the dignity of the one we care for and allowing love to be the driving force in all we do. When we love as He did, we reflect His heart—even in the smallest acts.

FOR THOUGHT:

In what ways has caregiving changed or deepened the way you understand love? How is God strengthening you to love with endurance—even when it's hard?

Take a moment to journal and share your heart with God.
Be open and honest, He can handle it.

PRAYER:

Jesus, thank You for loving me fully and faithfully. You never stop caring, even when I fall short. Help me to love like You—with patience, grace, and unwavering commitment. Strengthen me when I feel weak, and remind me that You are with me in every moment of caregiving. Let my love reflect Yours so that the one I care for can feel Your kindness through my hands. Teach me to love to the very end, just as You have loved me. Amen.

The Compassion of the Caregiver

"When he saw the crowds, he had compassion on them because they were confused and helpless, like sheep without a shepherd." Matthew 9:36 NLT

Jesus saw people—not just their needs, but their hearts. He didn't rush past their pain or fix them from a distance. He looked into their eyes, felt their burden, and responded with compassion.

This is the soul of caregiving: compassion that moves us to action. You do this every day. You see what others don't. You anticipate needs, ease fear, calm confusion, and give comfort—often without recognition or rest. That is the heart of Jesus living through you.

But let's be honest: compassion costs something. It can wear you down. It can make your heart feel raw. Sometimes, you may feel more like one of the "harassed and helpless" than the helper.

The good news? Jesus sees you too. And He has compassion for you. **You are not forgotten.** You are not carrying this alone. The same Shepherd who looked on the crowds with love looks on you with tenderness, care, and deep understanding.

So take a breath. Let His compassion cover you today—even as you pour it out for others.

FOR THOUGHT:

What does compassion look like in your daily caregiving—especially when you're tired or frustrated? How does it comfort you to know that Jesus sees and feels for both you and the one you care for?

Hey Caregiver
KEEP GOING

3

Take a moment to journal and share your heart with God.
Be open and honest, He can handle it.

....
....
....
....
....
....
....
....
....
....
....
....
....
....
....

PRAYER:

Jesus, You didn't look away from pain—you leaned into it with compassion. Teach me to see like You. Soften my heart when I'm tempted to harden it. Give me eyes to see the person behind the symptoms, and the strength to respond with love. And when I feel like the one who's worn down, remind me that You see me too. Thank You for caring for my soul as I care for someone else's. Shepherd me as I walk this journey. Amen.

Never Alone

"Teach these new disciples to obey all the commands I have given you. And be sure of this: I am with you always, even to the end of the age."
Matthew 28:20 NLT

Caregiving can be incredibly isolating. You might go hours—or even days—without a meaningful conversation. You may sit beside someone who doesn't recognize you anymore. You may feel invisible while doing work that rarely gets noticed.

But Jesus says something stunning: "I am with you—always."

Not just in the church pew.

Not just in your morning devotion.

Not just when things are going well.

But always—in the late-night hours, in the medication schedules, in the emotional exhaustion, and in the holy quiet of simply showing up.

Jesus is with you in the heavy lifting and the heartbreaking moments. He's there in the laughter, the tears, and the silences that say what words never could.

He is the God who stays.

This promise isn't temporary. It isn't conditional. It is eternal. And it's personal. Jesus isn't just near in some vague spiritual sense—He is with you. Holding you, guiding you, strengthening you, and never letting go.

You are never caregiving alone.

FOR THOUGHT:

Are there moments when you've doubted He was with you? What did you learn in those seasons? What comfort do you draw from knowing that Jesus' presence doesn't expire, fade, or withdraw?

Take a moment to journal and share your heart with God.
Be open and honest, He can handle it.

_____

_____

_____

_____

_____

_____

_____

_____

_____

_____

_____

_____

_____

PRAYER:

Jesus, thank You for the promise of Your presence. When I feel alone, remind me You are near. When I feel overwhelmed, steady me with Your peace. When no one else sees what I do, remind me that You do —and that You care deeply. Be my comfort in the quiet moments and my strength when I feel weak. Thank You for never leaving my side, even when I struggle. I trust that You are with me—now and always. Amen.

The Patient Love of Jesus

"Love is patient and kind. Love is not jealous or boastful or proud."
I Corinthians 13:4 NLT

Jesus' love is never rushed. He doesn't grow weary of us, even when we stumble over the same struggles or return to Him with the same tears. His patience is not reluctant tolerance—it is active, compassionate presence.

As the ultimate caregiver, Jesus shows patience in ways that challenge our own:

- With His disciples, when they didn't understand.
- With the crowds, when they interrupted His rest.
- With the sick, when they reached for healing.
- With Peter, when he denied Him—and Jesus restored him with grace.

He walks with us at our pace. He waits for us without shame. He tends to us in love that does not push, pressure, or punish. That's the kind of caregiver He is. And that's the kind of caregiver He empowers you to be.

In your own role, patience may be tested by repeated questions, unexpected messes, or long days with little change. But Jesus invites you not only to show patience—He invites you to receive it.

You're not failing when you feel frustrated. You're human. And Jesus—the One who never tires of loving you—offers His steady presence so you can love with the same grace He gives you daily.

Let His patient love fill you today… and let it spill over into your caregiving.

FOR THOUGHT:

When have you seen patience make the biggest difference in a caregiving moment? How did that reflect the heart of Jesus?

7

Take a moment to journal and share your heart with God.
Be open and honest, He can handle it.

_____

_____

_____

_____

_____

_____

_____

_____

_____

_____

_____

_____

_____

_____

PRAYER:

Jesus, thank You for being endlessly patient with me. When I'm slow to learn, when I fall short, or when I feel tired and stretched thin— You never walk away. Teach me to care for others with that same spirit. When I'm tempted to rush, remind me to pause. When I'm frustrated, whisper peace to my soul. Help me to see through Your eyes and love with Your heart. Thank You for caring for me gently, patiently, and without fail. Amen.

Gentle Strength in the Weary

"A bruised reed shall he not break, and smoking flax shall he not quench, till he send forth judgment unto victory." Matthew 12:20 KJV

Caregiving often stretches us beyond what we thought we could bear. Sometimes, you may feel bruised—fragile, worn, and vulnerable. Other times, your inner flame of hope or joy may feel like it's barely flickering.

But Jesus sees you in these moments. He does not break the bruised reed. He does not snuff out the smoldering wick. Instead, He draws near with gentle hands and patient heart. He protects what little strength you have left and nurtures your spirit to keep going.

This verse is a promise that you are not alone or forgotten in your weariness. Jesus is tender with your fragility and will not abandon you until His justice and healing come through fully.

In your caregiving, when patience runs thin and hope feels distant, rest in His gentle strength. Let Him tend your heart as you tend to others. Know that your faithfulness, no matter how small it seems, is part of a greater victory that He is bringing about.

FOR THOUGHT:

In what ways do you feel "bruised" in your caregiver journey— emotionally, mentally, or spiritually?

Hey Caregiver
KEEP PUSHING.

Take a moment to journal and share your heart with God.
Be open and honest, He can handle it.

Lord Jesus, I come to You feeling bruised and tired. Sometimes I wonder if I can keep going. But Your promise that You will not break the fragile parts of me brings me comfort. You cherish my weak places and keep my flame from going out. Help me to trust You more deeply—to lean on Your gentle strength when I feel worn. Restore my heart and renew my hope so I can continue caring with love and grace. Thank You for never leaving me alone in this journey. Amen.

Jesus Sees Your Heart

"Jesus knew what they were thinking, so he asked them, "Why do you question this in your hearts?" Luke 5:22 NIV

Caregiving is a journey filled with complex emotions—love, exhaustion, hope, frustration, guilt, and sometimes even doubt. Many times, the heaviest burdens we carry aren't just physical but hidden in the quiet corners of our hearts where thoughts swirl and feelings settle.

Jesus knows these inner thoughts. He sees beyond the surface and understands the struggles that no one else may fully grasp. He asks gently—not to condemn—but to bring what's hidden into the light where healing can begin.

You don't have to hide your true feelings from Him. You don't have to pretend everything is okay when it isn't. Jesus invites you to be honest and vulnerable, knowing that His love and forgiveness embrace you fully.

In this openness, there is freedom. The freedom to let go of guilt, the freedom to receive grace, and the freedom to continue your caregiving with renewed strength and peace.

FOR THOUGHT:

What are some thoughts or feelings you've been hesitant to admit—even to yourself—during this caregiving journey? What steps can you take to nurture honesty and healing in your heart and mind as you continue caring for your loved one?

Hey Caregiver

KEEP PUSHING.

11

Take a moment to journal and share your heart with God.
Be open and honest, He can handle it.

···
···
···
···
···
···
···
···
···
···
···
···
···
···

PRAYER:

Lord Jesus, You know the deepest thoughts and feelings I keep inside.
Sometimes I'm afraid to bring them to light because I fear judgment
or shame. But You ask with love and invite me into freedom. Help
me to be honest with You today—about my doubts, my fears, and my
frustrations. Thank You for Your unconditional love and forgiveness.
Heal my heart and give me strength to continue caring with grace.
Remind me that You see me, You know me, and You are always with
me. Amen.

Following the Example of Jesus

"I have given you an example to follow. Do as I have done to you."
John 13:15 NLT

Jesus knew He was about to face the cross. Yet, in one of His final acts before that moment, He knelt to wash His disciples' feet—dusty, tired feet that had walked with Him, questioned Him, even doubted Him. He didn't demand recognition. He chose humble service. Why? Because He wanted to show what love looks like in action.

As a caregiver, you are living that example—day in and day out.

When you bathe your loved one, when you feed them, comfort them, speak gently to them—you are embodying the same love that knelt low in the upper room. What you do may not look glamorous, and it often goes unseen, but in God's kingdom, serving is never small.

Jesus' example wasn't just about foot washing—it was about selfless love, patient presence, and the dignity of meeting someone's needs. And He doesn't just give you the command—He gives you His strength, His Spirit, and His smile.

Your caregiving is not just a duty. It's a holy imitation of the Savior.

FOR THOUGHT:

How can you reflect the heart of Jesus--His tenderness, attentiveness, and dignity—in the way your care for your loved one? What small, simple act of love could you do today that mirrors the spirit of foot-washing—personal, humble, and sacred?

**Take a moment to journal and share your heart with God.
Be open and honest, He can handle it.**

Lord Jesus, thank You for setting the example of humble love.
Sometimes caregiving is tiring, messy, and thankless—but You
remind me that no act of love is wasted. Help me to serve with Your
heart—with gentleness, patience, and grace. Give me strength on the
hard days and peace in the quiet moments. And when I feel unseen,
remind me that You see me. Let me love like You did, not for
recognition, but out of a heart full of Your Spirit. Amen.

Love That Stays

"Before the Passover celebration, Jesus knew that his hour had come to leave this world and return to his Father. He had loved his disciples during his ministry on earth, and now he loved them to the very end." John 13:1 NLT

Jesus knew His time on earth was drawing to a close. He had taught, healed, wept, and walked with His disciples—but now, with the cross ahead, He gathered them close. And Scripture tells us something breathtaking: He loved them to the end.

That's the kind of love that doesn't quit when it gets hard.

It doesn't walk away when it's unreturned or unrecognized.

It stays.

Caregiving is one of the clearest reflections of that kind of love. It's not always glamorous or applauded. It's often exhausting, and sometimes lonely. But each meal served, each diaper changed, each gentle word spoken is an act of enduring love—a love that chooses to remain, to give, to stay.

Jesus doesn't ask you to do this alone. He knows what it feels like to pour yourself out for others. He knows what it costs. And He promises that His Spirit is with you—giving you the strength to love beyond your limits.

You are not just surviving. You are participating in a holy echo of Jesus' love.

You are loving someone all the way to the end—and He sees it.

FOR THOUGHT:

Jesus didn't stop loving when it became hard—He leaned in. How can you draw closer to your loved one even when you feel weary? What does love require of you today?

15

Take a moment to journal and share your heart with God.
Be open and honest, He can handle it.

Jesus, thank You for loving so faithfully—without giving up or walking away. You see the long days and the quiet sacrifices I make as a caregiver. Some days I feel strong; other days I feel empty. Teach me to love like You—to stay present, to serve gently, and to hold nothing back. When I feel like I can't go further, fill me with Your strength. Let my caregiving be a reflection of Your unfailing love. Thank You for walking this road with me. Amen.

Ruth: Love That Stays

"But Ruth replied, 'Don't urge me to leave you or to turn back from you. Where you go I will go, and where you stay I will stay. Your people will be my people and your God my God.'" Ruth 1:16 NIV

Ruth's words are more than poetic—they are powerful. Spoken not in ease but in grief, her vow was forged in the fire of loss. She was a widow with no promises ahead, yet she chose to stay, to care, and to walk alongside her mother-in-law, Naomi, into an uncertain future.

This is the heart of a caregiver: not someone who always has answers, but someone who shows up, stays close, and says, "Where you go, I will go."

Caregiving often involves sacrifices—of time, dreams, routines, or even identity. But in the quiet acts of presence and love, God writes a greater story, just as He did with Ruth. Her faithfulness became the soil from which the lineage of Christ would grow.

As a caregiver, your daily faithfulness may feel unnoticed or ordinary, but it carries the weight of covenant love—one that reflects God's own steadfastness. The world may not see it, but Heaven does. You are walking in the footsteps of Ruth, and God is walking with you.

FOR THOUGHT:

In what ways do you relate to Ruth's decision to stay and walk alongside someone in need, no matter the cost? What do you need from God today to continue showing up with love, like Ruth, in the place you've been called to serve?

Hey Caregiver
KEEP LOVING.

Take a moment to journal and share your heart with God.
Be open and honest, He can handle it.

PRAYER:

Lord, thank You for Ruth's example of faithfulness and strength. In her choice to stay and serve, I see a reflection of my own caregiving journey—one filled with both sacrifice and purpose. Sometimes it's hard. Sometimes I feel like turning back. But You remind me that love stays, even when the road is unclear. Strengthen my spirit today. Help me to love not just with my hands, but with my heart. Let me serve with faith and courage, trusting that You are writing a bigger story through every small act. Amen.

The Good Samaritan: The Compassion That Stops

"But a Samaritan, as he traveled, came where the man was; and when he saw him, he took pity on him. He went to him and bandaged his wounds…"
Luke 10:33–34 NIV

The Good Samaritan didn't plan to be a caregiver that day. He was on a journey—minding his business, tending to his life. But then he saw someone in pain, and he stopped.

He could have passed by, like the others. Instead, he got close enough to see the wounds. He got involved. He gave his own supplies. He used his strength and resources to lift the broken and carry him to safety.

That is what caregivers do—every day.

You see the wounds others don't see. You respond with action when others walk away. You stop your own plans to bind up someone else's pain. And just like the Samaritan, you don't always get recognition—but you reflect the very heart of God.

Jesus told this story to show us what neighborly love looks like. But for caregivers, this is more than a story. It's your life. Your hands bind wounds, your time becomes healing, and your presence becomes a place of peace.

In a world that often passes by, you stop.

And that's sacred.

FOR THOUGHT:

How do you respond when caregiving interrupts your plans or expectations? What does this reveal about your willingness to serve like Jesus? What boundaries or self-care practices do you need to maintain so that you can continue caregiving with compassion rather than burnout?

PRAYER:

Jesus, thank You for the example of the Good Samaritan. Help me to love like he did—with eyes that see, a heart that feels, and hands that act. When I feel weary from caregiving, remind me that what I'm doing is holy work. Let compassion steady me when I'm tempted to rush or withdraw. Help me serve without needing applause. You see every wound I tend to, every interruption I embrace, and every sacrifice I make. Strengthen me to stop, to serve, and to love as You do. Amen.

Martha and Mary: The Balance of Doing and Being

"But Martha was distracted by all the preparations that had to be made. She came to him and asked, 'Lord, don't you care that my sister has left me to do the work by myself? Tell her to help me!'" Luke 10:40 NIV

Martha wasn't wrong for serving—she was showing love the best way she knew how. But Scripture tells us she was distracted. Her heart, though willing, was worn thin by responsibility.

Sound familiar?

Caregiving often puts us in Martha's shoes—tending, cooking, cleaning, assisting, arranging, advocating. It's beautiful work. But sometimes, even good work can leave us feeling unseen, exhausted, or even frustrated with those who don't seem to carry the same weight.

Jesus didn't scold Martha for working—He lovingly redirected her. He reminded her that service isn't just about doing—it's about being: being with Him, being still, and letting our soul breathe in His presence.

As caregivers, the most important thing you bring to your role isn't just your effort—it's your presence, grounded in God's peace. Like Mary, you're invited to sit, rest, and receive—even in the middle of a busy day.

Because caregiving is not just about how much you do—it's about staying connected to the One who strengthens you to do it.

FOR THOUGHT:

How can you better balance necessary caregiving duties with the nourishment of your own soul? What rhythms or boundaries need to shift? What does it look like to serve from a place of peace rather than pressure? What do you need from Jesus to begin doing that?

_____

_____

_____

_____

_____

_____

_____

_____

_____

_____

_____

_____

_____

PRAYER:

Jesus, You see me when I'm like Martha—working hard, trying to keep everything together, yet feeling stretched and unnoticed. Thank You for gently reminding me to pause and be with You. Help me find moments to sit at Your feet, even in a full day. Let my caregiving flow from a heart anchored in Your peace, not driven by pressure. Teach me to balance serving with stillness. And when I feel alone in the weight I carry, remind me that You are near, and I am never unseen. Amen.

Joseph: The Quiet Yes

"When Joseph woke up, he did as the angel of the Lord commanded and took Mary as his wife." Matthew 1:24 NLT

Joseph doesn't speak a single recorded word in Scripture, yet his life speaks volumes. One verse captures a moment of decision—he woke up, and he did what God asked of him. No resistance. No fanfare. Just quiet obedience in the face of enormous responsibility.

As a caregiver, you may resonate with Joseph more than you realize. You show up, often quietly. You adjust your life around someone else's needs. You may not get a lot of attention or thanks—but you carry out a sacred assignment with daily, consistent love.

Joseph accepted a calling that wasn't easy. He took on the weight of protection, provision, and care—because God entrusted him with someone vulnerable and important. So have you.

Your "yes" to caregiving might not have come through an angel in a dream, but it is no less holy. And God sees it. He honors it. Your obedience—your faithfulness in the day-to-day—is writing a story just as valuable as Joseph's: one of trust, courage, and love.

FOR THOUGHT:

What fears or doubts might Joseph have faced when stepping into this unexpected role? What fears do you wrestle with in your caregiving journey? How can you honor the quiet strength it takes to be a caregiver--especially when your role requires more sacrifice than spotlight?

Take a moment to journal and share your heart with God.
Be open and honest, He can handle it.

....
....
....
....
....
....
....
....
....
....
....
....
....
....

PRAYER:

God, thank You for Joseph—an example of obedience without applause. Thank You for showing me that faithfulness doesn't always need a spotlight to be significant. Sometimes I feel like my efforts go unnoticed, but You see every quiet act of love. Help me to serve with the same trust Joseph had. Renew my strength to keep saying yes each day—to keep showing up, even when it's hard. Remind me that my caregiving matters to You and that my quiet obedience brings glory to Your name. Amen.

The Women at the Cross: Faithful to the End

"Many women were there, watching from a distance. They had followed Jesus from Galilee to care for his needs." Matthew 27:55 NIV

They didn't run.

As Jesus suffered on the cross, many had already scattered—too afraid, too overwhelmed, too broken to stay. But the women remained. They stood at a distance, yes, but they stood with Him. These women had followed Jesus for a long time. They had cared for Him, served Him, and now, they stayed with Him—even when it cost them deeply.

This is the sacred strength of a caregiver.

Faithfulness doesn't always look like loud declarations or perfect strength. Sometimes it looks like standing quietly beside someone's pain. Sometimes it's found in holding a hand, making a meal, or staying near when others drift away.

As a caregiver, you embody this kind of love. Your quiet commitment, your willingness to keep showing up, your steady presence—these things reflect the same courageous devotion shown by the women at the cross. And just as Jesus saw them, He sees you.

Faithful caregiving isn't just about getting through it—it's about loving someone well, all the way through. And that, dear caregiver, is holy ground.

FOR THOUGHT:

The women stayed, even as others fled. What motivates you to stay when caregiving gets emotionally or spiritually overwhelming? What does this verse teach you about legacy—that even in quiet, faithful service, God remembers and honors those who love well?

Take a moment to journal and share your heart with God.
Be open and honest, He can handle it.

_____

_____

_____

_____

_____

_____

_____

_____

_____

_____

_____

_____

_____

_____

PRAYER:

Jesus, thank You for the women who stood near You in Your final hours. Thank You for their courage, their tenderness, and their steadfast love. I see my own journey in theirs—walking beside someone in pain, offering care that often goes unseen. Lord, help me to be faithful to the end. When I feel weary, strengthen me. When I feel invisible, remind me that You see me. Teach me how to love without fear, and to remain present, even when the load is heavy. Let my caregiving reflect the same love You showed on the cross—faithful, sacrificial, and unshakable. Amen.

Strength for the Journey

"So let's not get tired of doing what is good. At just the right time we will reap a harvest of blessing if we don't give up." Galatians 6:9 NLT

Caregiving is one of the most sacred and selfless acts of love, yet it often goes unseen and uncelebrated. Days blur together, progress can be slow, and the weight of responsibility feels endless. In Galatians 6:9, God speaks directly into this space of fatigue and faithfulness: *"Let us not get tired of doing what is good. At just the right time, we will reap a harvest of blessing if we don't give up."*

God sees every act of love you pour out—every meal prepared, every tear wiped, every prayer whispered in the quiet. While the world may not applaud you, heaven is paying attention. The "harvest" may not come all at once, and it may not look like what you expect. But it will come—in strength, in spiritual depth, in moments of grace, and ultimately, in God's eternal reward.

You are not forgotten. You are sowing seeds of eternal significance.

FOR THOUGHT:

When do you feel most tired or discouraged in doing good in your caregiving role? How can you invite God into the moments when you feel like quitting?

Hey Caregiver

KEEP CARING

Take a moment to journal and share your heart with God.
Be open and honest, He can handle it.

PRAYER:

Father, you see me when no one else does. You know the strength it takes to care, to serve, and to keep showing up. On the days when I feel worn down, remind me that what I'm doing matters—not just to the one I care for, but to You. Give me endurance for today and hope for tomorrow. Let me trust that the seeds I plant in love will one day grow into something beautiful. Help me not to give up, because You never give up on me. In Jesus' name, Amen.

Strength for the Silent Battle

"So do not fear, for I am with you... I will strengthen you and help you."
Isaiah 41:10 NIV

Caregiving can often feel like a silent battle—one that drains your energy, tests your patience, and sometimes leaves you feeling unseen and alone. But God breaks into that silence with a steady, loving voice: "So do not fear, for I am with you... I will strengthen you and help you."

God doesn't promise a pain-free path, but He does promise His presence. You don't have to face the exhaustion, the hard decisions, or the emotional weight by yourself. You don't have to carry the fear of what's ahead, because the One who holds the future is holding you.

When your hands are full and your heart is tired, He is your strength. When you don't have the answers, He is your help. When you feel like no one sees the sacrifices you make—He sees. And He honors your faithfulness more than you know.

Let this verse be your anchor. Not a suggestion to try harder, but a divine promise: You are not alone.

FOR THOUGHT:

What fears are you carrying in this caregiving season? What do you need to surrender so you can receive God's strength instead of just relying on your own?

Hey Caregiver
MORE GRACE

....

....

....

....

....

....

....

....

....

....

....

....

....

....

PRAYER:

Father, thank You for being with me, even when I feel like I'm running on empty. In the moments when fear creeps in and I feel overwhelmed, remind me that You are my God, and You are near. Strengthen me when I'm weak. Help me when I don't know what to do. Teach me to rely on Your power, not just my own effort. And above all, wrap me in the comfort of Your presence. I may not have control over everything, but I trust the One who holds me. In Jesus' name, Amen.

Strength Beyond Your Own

"I can do all things through Christ who strengthens me." Philippians 4:13 NKJV

Caregiving stretches you in ways you never imagined. Some days feel manageable. Other days feel like survival. But in Philippians 4:13, Paul reminds us of something radical: *"I can do all things through Christ who strengthens me."*

This verse doesn't mean you have to do everything perfectly, nor does it promise a life without exhaustion or struggle. It means that whatever you're called to do—whether it's helping your loved one through another difficult night, making a hard decision, or facing yet another day with no thanks or rest—you're not doing it alone.

God's strength shows up in your smallest faithful acts: when you stay instead of walk away, when you speak gently though you feel frayed, when you rise again after crying in secret.

You're not expected to be strong—only to lean on the One who is.

Caregiving through Christ means surrender, trust, and allowing His grace to hold you up when you don't think you can go on. And He will.

FOR THOUGHT:

What does "all things" mean to you as a caregiver? Are there limits you've placed on yourself or on God? How can you more intentionally invite Jesus into your caregiving moments?

Hey Caregiver
GOD'S GOT YOU.

31

PRAYER:

Lord Jesus, You know how tired I am. Some days I don't feel strong enough to do this. Thank You for the promise that I don't have to rely on my strength alone. Remind me that You are with me, working through me, and giving me what I need each day. Help me to pause, breathe, and remember: I can do all things through You—especially the hard things. Help me to trust that You're not just beside me, but within me. Strengthen my heart, my hands, and my hope. In Your name I pray, Amen.

The Gift of Rest

"Come to Me, all who are weary and burdened, and I will give you rest."
Matthew 11:28 NIV

Caregiving is sacred work, but it can also be relentless. The constant need, the emotional highs and lows, the physical toll—it can leave you feeling bone-weary and unseen. Into this reality, Jesus gently speaks: *"Come to Me, all who are weary and burdened, and I will give you rest."*

He doesn't offer a quick fix. He doesn't promise to remove the caregiving responsibilities. But He does promise something even deeper: soul rest. Rest that goes beyond sleep or a break. Rest that calms the storm inside and steadies your spirit.

Jesus invites you to trade your heavy yoke of "I have to do it all" for His yoke of love, gentleness, and grace. His yoke doesn't remove effort—it just shifts the weight. You're not carrying it alone anymore.

When you feel invisible, exhausted, or stretched beyond your limits, remember: Jesus sees you. And He doesn't ask you to be stronger—He asks you to come closer. To learn from Him. To breathe. To rest in His steady presence.

You're not failing because you're tired. You're human. And He's offering you peace.

FOR THOUGHT:

What burdens are you carrying that you haven't fully brought to Jesus? What would change if you truly trusted Jesus to carry this with you?

Hey Caregiver
YOU ARE AMAZING

Take a moment to journal and share your heart with God.
Be open and honest, He can handle it.

Jesus, I come to You tired and stretched thin. I've been carrying so much—responsibility, fear, grief, guilt. But You invite me to lay it all down and take up Your rest. Teach me to walk with You at a slower, gentler pace. Help me to stop striving and start trusting. Remind me that You are with me, carrying this burden alongside me. Even when the demands don't change, let my heart be changed by Your peace. I receive Your rest today—not just for my body, but for my soul. In Your faithful name I pray, Amen.

Peace That Stays

"I am leaving you with a gift—peace of mind and heart. And the peace I give is a gift the world cannot give. So don't be troubled or afraid." John 14:27 NLT

Caregiving can be a constant storm of responsibilities, emotions, and uncertainty. In the middle of it all, Jesus offers a calm anchor for the soul: *"Peace I leave with you; my peace I give you. I do not give to you as the world gives..."*

The world's peace is often temporary—dependent on circumstances. A moment of quiet, a rare full night of sleep, a good report from the doctor. But Jesus promises a different kind of peace —a peace that stays. It's not based on what's happening around you, but on Who is with you.

His peace meets you in the hospital waiting room. In the middle of the night when you're exhausted. In the moments when you're afraid of what tomorrow will bring.

Jesus doesn't ask you to pretend you're not tired or troubled. He just invites you to trade the heaviness of fear for the security of His presence.

You don't have to fix everything. You don't have to hold everything together. He is holding you. And His peace is not fragile. It's a gift. Receive it.

FOR THOUGHT:

What thoughts or fears do you rehearse that steal your peace? How would it change your day to hand over those troubles in prayer each morning? How can you practice courage through trust in Jesus today?

PRAYER:

Jesus, thank You for offering me peace that is deeper than my circumstances. You see how heavy my heart can get—how fear and stress sometimes take over. Today, I choose to receive Your peace. Let it quiet my racing thoughts and ease the tension in my soul. Help me not to chase the world's version of relief, but to rest in what You've already given. Even when I'm surrounded by uncertainty, let Your peace be the most real thing I know. Be my calm in the storm. I trust You. In Your name I pray, Amen.

Where Your Help Comes From

"I will lift up mine eyes unto the hills, from whence cometh my help. My help cometh from the Lord, which made heaven and earth." Psalm 121:1-2 KJV

There are days in caregiving when the weight feels unbearable—emotionally, physically, spiritually. You do what needs to be done, but deep down, you're asking the same quiet question the psalmist did: *"Where does my help come from?"*

Psalm 121 doesn't just ask that question—it answers it with power and peace: *"My help comes from the Lord, the Maker of heaven and earth."*

It's not a distant, indifferent God who helps you. It's the Creator —the One who sculpted the mountains you're staring up at. The One who knows your every burden, sees your unseen labor, and supplies strength when yours runs out.

He doesn't just offer help; He is your help. You don't have to carry this alone. You're not expected to be the savior in this story. That job is already taken. Your job is to lift your eyes—to remember where your help truly comes from.

Even on the hardest days, when you feel like you're barely holding it together, God is holding you.

FOR THOUGHT:

Have you invited God into the moments where you most need help, or have you been trying to manage on your own? What does trusting God as your helper look like in the daily details of caregiving?

Take a moment to journal and share your heart with God.
Be open and honest, He can handle it.

God, some days I don't even know where to look for help. The weight of caregiving is more than I can carry on my own. But You remind me to lift my eyes—not to my worries, not to my own strength, but to You. You are my Helper. You made the heavens and the earth, and You see me. You care for me. You will not let me fall. Give me the faith to lift my eyes to You today. Help me feel Your presence, Your power, and Your peace. In Jesus' name, Amen.

Grace in the Cracks

"Each time he said, "My grace is all you need. My power works best in weakness. So now I am glad to boast about my weaknesses, so that the power of Christ can work through me." 2 Corinthians 12:9 NLT

Caregiving has a way of exposing your limits—physically, emotionally, mentally, and spiritually. You may find yourself saying, "I can't do this anymore," or "I'm not strong enough for this." But in 2 Corinthians 12:9, God gently speaks into those cracks: *"My grace is sufficient for you, for my power is made perfect in weakness."*

This verse doesn't shame you for feeling weak—it celebrates it. God's strength doesn't require your perfection. His grace doesn't wait for you to have it all together. In fact, it meets you right where you're falling apart.

What if your breaking point is actually a meeting point—with the God who never runs out of patience, love, or power?

You were never meant to do this in your own strength. The pressure to be strong for everyone else is heavy, but it was never yours to carry alone. When you allow yourself to be vulnerable before God, you open the door for His power to rest on you—not just to help you survive, but to strengthen you in soul-deep, lasting ways.

God is not asking you to fake it. He's asking you to lean in.

FOR THOUGHT:

What would change if you believed that God's power shines most brightly through your limitations? What would it look like for you to carry out your caregiving with Christ's power instead of your own?

_____

_____

_____

_____

_____

_____

_____

_____

_____

_____

_____

_____

_____

_____

_____

PRAYER:

Lord, I feel my weaknesses every day—my exhaustion, my impatience, my doubts. But You tell me that Your grace is enough. That Your power shines through the very places I try to hide. Help me stop pretending I'm strong and start trusting that You are. Let Your strength rest on me—not just to get through the day, but to be changed by Your presence in it. Teach me to boast in my weakness because that's where I find You most. In Jesus' name, Amen.

Hope That Overflows

"May the God of hope fill you with all joy and peace as you trust in him, so that you may overflow with hope by the power of the Holy Spirit."
Romans 15:13 NIV

Caregiving often feels like pouring from an empty cup. You're constantly giving—time, energy, compassion—sometimes without rest, without thanks, and without much left for yourself. But Romans 15:13 reminds us that hope, joy, and peace aren't things we have to manufacture. They're gifts from God—meant to fill us, not just visit us.

The hope God gives isn't based on outcomes. It's rooted in who He is. He is the God of hope—not scarcity, not burnout, not disappointment. And when you trust in Him, even imperfectly, He promises to fill you.

Joy and peace may not erase the exhaustion or the pain—but they soften it. They become quiet companions, reminding you that you are not alone. And when the Holy Spirit moves in you, what once felt like emptiness can become overflow—hope spilling out from a heart that has been filled by grace.

So when you feel drained, defeated, or unseen, don't try harder—receive. Trust. Let Him fill the spaces you can't fill on your own.

FOR THOUGHT:

What does hope look like for you in this caregiving season? Are you trying to do this caregiving journey on your own strength, or leaning on the Holy Spirit?

Hey Caregiver

HEAVEN SEES

PRAYER:

God of hope, I need You. I'm tired of trying to carry everything alone. Please fill me today—not just with energy, but with joy and peace that only come from trusting You. Help me to stop relying on my own strength and to start leaning into Yours. Let Your Spirit breathe fresh hope into my heart, even when circumstances stay the same. Teach me to live not from survival, but from the overflow of Your presence. In Jesus' name, Amen.

The Promise That Holds You

He will wipe every tear from their eyes, and there will be no more death or sorrow or crying or pain. All these things are gone forever."
Revelation 21:4 NLT

Caregiving can feel like a slow kind of grief—watching someone you love change, decline, or slip away piece by piece. There are tears no one sees. Pain that can't always be explained. And deep mourning over things that used to be simple.

But God sees it all. And in Revelation 21:4, He gives a breathtaking promise: *"He will wipe every tear from their eyes. There will be no more death or mourning or crying or pain..."*

This is not poetic language—it is personal comfort. God Himself will wipe your tears. Not just stop them. Wipe them. Gently. Tenderly. As only someone who truly cares would do.

He promises a day when everything you've carried will be lifted. When death, dementia, sorrow, and sickness will be undone. A day when caregiving will no longer be needed—because healing will be complete.

But even now—before that day comes—God is not distant. He draws near to the brokenhearted. He holds every tear in His hands. And when you feel like you can't go on, He reminds you:
This is not the end of the story.

You are part of something eternal. And every loving act you offer now is not forgotten—it's treasured by the One who will one day restore all things.

FOR THOUGHT:

What tears have you shed in this caregiving season that feel unseen or unacknowledged? What would it look like to invite God into those places?

PRAYER:

God, sometimes this journey is heavy with pain and silent sorrow. Thank You for the promise that You see every tear I cry, and that one day You will wipe them all away. Help me hold on to that hope when today feels too much. Teach me to live with eternity in mind, trusting that this pain is not forever. Comfort me now as I wait for the world You are making new. Thank You for being near, even in the grief. In Jesus' name, Amen.

Held When Things Fall Apart

"God is our refuge and strength, an ever-present help in trouble. Therefore we will not fear, though the earth give way and the mountains fall into the heart of the sea." Psalm 46:1-2 NIV

Caregiving often means living in the middle of chaos—doctors' appointments, changing symptoms, emotional highs and lows. Sometimes it feels like the ground beneath you is crumbling. Plans collapse. Strength fades. Hope thins out.

But Psalm 46:1–2 offers a steady hand in the storm: *"God is our refuge and strength, an ever-present help in trouble. Therefore we will not fear, though the earth give way..."*

God doesn't promise to remove the trouble, but He does promise to be right in it with you. Not distant. Not delayed. Ever-present. When everything around you feels unstable, He is your refuge—your safe shelter. He is your strength—your energy when you have none. He is your help—your wisdom when you don't know what to do next.

Even if your world feels like it's falling apart, you are not falling apart—because God is holding you.

You don't have to carry the fear. You don't have to hold it all together. He already is.

FOR THOUGHT:

When was the last time you truly allowed God to be your refuge-- your safe place? What would it look like today to rest in God as both your shelter and your source?

_____

_____

_____

_____

_____

_____

_____

_____

_____

_____

_____

_____

_____

_____

PRAYER:

God, some days I feel like the ground beneath me is shaking. So much is uncertain, and I'm so tired of trying to be strong. Thank You for being my refuge when life is too much. Thank You for being my strength when I have nothing left to give. Remind me that You are not far off—you are right here with me. I bring You my fear, my fatigue, and my fractured heart. Hold me steady today. I trust You to carry what I cannot. In Jesus' name, Amen.

A Love That Keeps Showing Up

"Love is patient, love is kind. It does not envy, it does not boast, it is not proud. It does not dishonor others, it is not self-seeking, it is not easily angered, it keeps no record of wrongs. Love does not delight in evil but rejoices with the truth. It always protects, always trusts, always hopes, always perseveres."
1 Corinthians 13:4-7 NIV

Caregiving is one of the purest forms of love—and one of the most exhausting. It's love that shows up when it's not convenient. It gives when nothing is given back. It often goes unseen, unthanked, and uncelebrated.

In 1 Corinthians 13:4–7, we find a definition of love that speaks directly to the kind of love caregiving requires: *"Love is patient, love is kind… It always protects, always trusts, always hopes, always perseveres."*

This is not surface love. This is sacrificial, persevering, gritty love —the kind that folds laundry at midnight, holds trembling hands, answers repeated questions without anger, and fights to maintain dignity when disease tries to steal it.

But let's be honest: sometimes this kind of love feels impossible.

That's because this love isn't something we muster—it's something we receive and reflect. It starts with God's love for us. He is patient with you. He is kind to you. He never keeps a record of your wrongs. And when you're at the end of yourself, His love is what refuels you to go another day.

You don't have to love perfectly. You just have to stay connected to the One who does.

FOR THOUGHT:

In what areas of caregiving is it hardest for you to remain patient? How might forgiveness free you—not just them—from emotional weight?

PRAYER:

God, thank You for loving me with a love that never runs out. Some days, caregiving stretches me past my patience and into my breaking point. I confess the times I've been short, bitter, or weary of doing good. Thank You for meeting me in those places with grace, not guilt. Fill me with Your love so that I can pour it out freely. Help me love with kindness, humility, and perseverance—not from my own strength, but from Yours. Remind me that when I love like You, I reflect Your heart. In Jesus' name, Amen.

What You Wear Matters

*"Since God chose you to be the holy people he loves, you must clothe yourselves
with tenderhearted mercy, kindness, humility, gentleness, and patience. Make
allowance for each other's faults, and forgive anyone who offends you. Remember,
the Lord forgave you, so you must forgive others. Colossians 3:12-13 NLT*

Caregiving is more than a list of tasks—it's an emotional and
spiritual calling that pulls on every part of you. Some days you wake
up with a full heart. Other days, you're already tired before your feet
hit the floor. On those days, this passage from Colossians becomes
more than a suggestion—it becomes a lifeline: *"Clothe yourselves
with compassion, kindness, humility, gentleness and patience... Bear
with each other and forgive..."*

God isn't asking you to summon these things on your own. He's
inviting you to put them on like clothing—deliberately, daily,
intentionally. Just as you get dressed each morning, you have the
chance to wrap yourself in what reflects His heart.

It doesn't mean you won't feel frustration, grief, or exhaustion. It
means when you do, there's something stronger you can reach for:
His grace, His presence, His character at work in you.

And when others fail you—family members who don't help,
friends who don't understand, even the one you're caring for who
might lash out in confusion or pain—God reminds you: Forgive as I
have forgiven you.

That kind of forgiveness doesn't deny the hurt. It simply refuses to
let it harden your heart.

You're not alone in this. You're not unequipped. You are chosen,
holy, and dearly loved. And you're never expected to do this without
Him.

What would it look like to consciously "clothe yourself" with compassion before starting each caregiving day? What situations or behaviors test your ability to "bear with" your loved one right now?

Hey Caregiver

GOD HONORS YOU.

PRAYER:

Lord, You see the weight I carry and the emotions I wrestle with. Some days it's hard to be kind. Some moments, I run out of patience. But You remind me that I am dearly loved—and from that love, I can draw strength. Help me clothe myself with compassion and humility, not because I feel like it, but because You live in me. Teach me how to forgive freely, as You have forgiven me. And when I fall short, gently help me try again. Thank You for never leaving me to do this alone. In Jesus' name, Amen.

Give What You Can, Not What You Don't Have

"Do not withhold good from those who deserve it when it's in your power to help them." Proverbs 3:27 NLT

Caregiving often feels like a constant giving of yourself—your time, your strength, your emotions. Some days you give willingly. Other days, you give wearily. And then there are moments you wonder if you have anything left to give at all.

In Proverbs 3:27, we're told: *"Do not withhold good from those to whom it is due, when it is in your power to act."*

This verse isn't a command to exhaust yourself. It's not asking you to pour from an empty cup. Instead, it gently calls you to give what is within your power—not more, not less. Just what you honestly can.

God isn't measuring your caregiving by perfection or performance. He sees the small, sacred choices: the gentle tone when you're frustrated, the patience to repeat something one more time, the silent prayer when you feel invisible.

Sometimes "doing good" is a soft word. Sometimes it's showing up when you'd rather walk away. And sometimes, doing good means resting, so you have something left to give tomorrow.

This verse reminds us that goodness isn't about grand gestures—it's about being faithful with what's in your hands today.

Hey Caregiver
HANG IN THERE

How do you view the person you care for—as a burden, a duty, or someone worthy of honor or dignity? Have you unintentionally held back love, patience, or kindness because of exhaustion, resentment, or discouragement? How might you begin to offer "good" again, even in small and sustainable ways?

Hey Caregiver
YOU ROCK.

PRAYER:

Lord, You know how much I'm carrying. Sometimes I feel like I have nothing left to give. Thank You for reminding me that You don't expect more than what's in my power to give. Show me what "doing good" looks like today—help me offer love without resentment, serve with grace, and rest when needed. Remind me that every small act of care matters to You. Teach me to give freely but also wisely, trusting that You will fill me as I pour out. In Jesus' name, Amen.

God Never Forgets

"For God is not unjust. He will not forget how hard you have worked for him and how you have shown your love to him by caring for other believers, as you still do." Hebrews 6:10 NLT

One of the hardest things about caregiving is how invisible it can feel. You do so much behind the scenes—washing, lifting, listening, calming, comforting—and there's often no applause, no acknowledgment, no break. It can leave you wondering: Does anyone even see what I'm doing?

Hebrews 6:10 offers this quiet but powerful reassurance: *"God is not unjust; he will not forget your work and the love you have shown him as you have helped his people and continue to help them."*

God sees what no one else sees. Every sleepless night. Every act of patience. Every whispered prayer when you feel like giving up. None of it is wasted. None of it is forgotten.

And maybe even more comforting than that—He sees the love behind your care. Even if your loved one can't say thank you… even if family doesn't understand… even if you're running on fumes—God knows.

You're not just helping someone. You're honoring God through your help. You are loving Him by loving them.

So today, even if no one else notices—God does. And in His eyes, what you're doing is holy work.

What specific act of caregiving have you done recently that you need to remind yourself *God won't forget?* How can you begin to see your daily tasks not as chores, but as ministry? How does your care for your loved one become an expression of love to God?

Hey Caregiver

THANK YOU.

God, thank You for reminding me that You see me. When I feel invisible, underappreciated, or exhausted, help me remember that You never forget my work. You know how I pour myself out in love —and that matters to You. Strengthen me today. Fill me again with quiet confidence that my caregiving is not in vain. Help me see each act of service as an offering to You. And when I'm weary, whisper this truth back to my heart: You notice. You care. You are with me. In Jesus' name, Amen.

Journal

If it concerns you, it concerns God.

MY FAVORITE GIRL
CAREGIVERS CORNER
WITH PRISCILLA J. JEAN-LOUIS
PODCAST

PODCAST MISSION

Bringing inspiration, education, resources, and strength to Caregivers so you can **Keep Going. Keep Pushing. Keep Loving.** *Keep Caring.*

SUBSCRIBE

@My Favorite Girl
Caregivers Corner Podcast

FOLLOW

@My Favorite Girl & Alzheimer's

@MyFavoriteGirlandAlz

Priscilla Jean-Louis

www.priscillajjean-louis.com

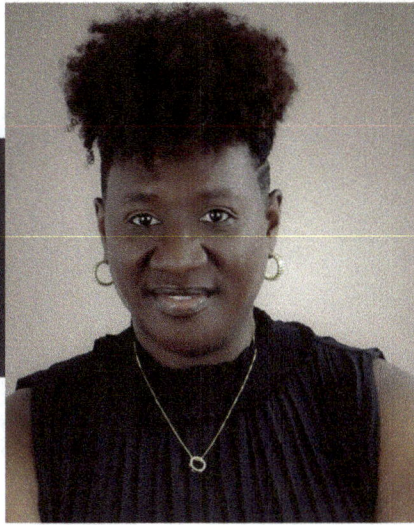

About the Author

PRISCILLA JEAN-LOUIS is an author, an ambassador of servant leadership, an inspirational caregiver and podcaster for family caregivers. In 2017, she became the primary caregiver for her mother who lives with Alzheimer's dementia. Subsequently in April 2018, she also took on caring for her grandmother who also lived with the disease. Priscilla is a relentless advocate for those who suffer from dementia and Alzheimer's and provides empathetic inspiration for their caregivers. Her response to God's mandate to make MINISTRY out of the MOMENTS was an emphatic "YES!"; and as a result, Priscilla took those ministry moments and created the social media platform, #MyFavoriteGirl & Alzheimer's and the My Favorite Girl Caregivers Corner Podcast to authentically, creatively, and humorously chronicle their journey and empower others to share their own.